# Diary of a Mad Lupus Patient

## Shortness of Breath

Written by J. H. JOHNSON

Edited by Alana D. MousaviDin

Diary of a Mad Lupus Patient: Shortness of Breath

Copyright © 2012 by J. H. Johnson

All rights reserved. This book or any portion thereof may not be reproduced or used in any manner whatsoever without the express written permission of the publisher except for the use of brief quotations in a book review.

The medical information in this book is provided without any representations or warranties, expressed or implied.

You must not rely on the information in this book as an alternative to medical advice from your doctor or other professional healthcare provider.

Printed in the United States of America
Published by Unique Variety Sales LLC
www.uniquevarietysales.com
First Printing, 2012
ISBN: 0988881055
ISBN-13: 978-0-9888810-5-1

Diary of a MAD Lupus Patient     J. H. Johnson

## **DEDICATION**

This book is dedicated to my mother who never saw me as sick and unable. She prayed for me to be well and able to do everything that she couldn't. Mama, I can do whatever I want because of you.

## ACKNOWLEDGMENTS

Acknowledgments are for those who know what they mean to me. To my husband Glenn, thank you for coming into my life. Thank you to my aunt Esther and my beloved mother, Hettie Ann. Thank you to Brandi, my pride and encouragement in many aspects of my personal life and career. A heartfelt "thank you," goes to my best friend Carmen, for her patience and endless laughter.

A very special thanks to Shawn, my sister and friend, who had the courage to accept my illness as it was from the very beginning. Thank you for walking to my house almost every day afterschool to keep me updated on the latest high school gossip. Thank you to all who helped me complete this project, kept me in good health, cheered my next steps, and provided the best care and personal support possible. Thank you to all of the women in my life that took the time to care and share. Thank you to Mrs. Beverly Clyburn, Mrs. Marion Gary, and Dr. Eavon Hickson for your encouragement, time, and support through the years. You touched my life and I grew. Dr. Hickson, thank you for taking the time to provide "love" edits where I needed them most.

And last, but not least, I want to thank my physicians, nurses, and friends who encouraged me to live and move forward. Thank you to all of my physicians for their patience and care. God is magnificent– I thank Him for giving me a gift of knowing who is best to cross my path in life.

Through God, all things are possible.

*"I can do all things through Christ which strengtheneth me."*
*~ Philippians 4:13 (King James Version)*

Diary of a MAD Lupus Patient　　　　　　J. H. Johnson

## PREFACE

This book is a re-write of a handwritten little notebook that was used to record medication changes, thoughts, feelings, pain, hurt, treatments, and the end of the world as I saw it when I was first diagnosed. Simply put, these pages compose the exact notes of my experiences upon the onset of systemic lupus erythematosus (SLE). Names have been changed to protect the privacy of others.

According to the Lupus Foundation of America, lupus is defined as a chronic, autoimmune disease that can damage any part of the body (skin, joints, and/or organs inside the body). The body's immune system produces auto-antibodies that attack healthy tissue and cause inflammation, pain, and damage in various parts of the body. At the time this diary was written, lupus was considered life threatening and incurable. At the time this diary was prepared in traditional book format, lupus was still considered a life threatening illness. There is still no cure for the disease.

Many symptoms affect those diagnosed with lupus in different ways. Lupus can affect several major organs of the body to include the brain, central nervous system, and the digestive system. Often called SLE by medical practitioners, lupus is known for creating a skin rash in the form of a butterfly. Forms of lupus vary and may include varying symptoms such as: chronic fatigue, fever, mouth sores, loss of hair, sensitivity to sunlight, and depression.

More information about the wide range of symptoms, forms, and treatments for Lupus can be found at http://www.lupus.org.

## INTRODUCTION

"Am I dead yet? Well, dang! The doctor lied! The doctors said that I wasn't going to make it ten years. Yet, here I am and still kicking. What is it that they say? It ain't over until it's over!" I must admit, in the beginning, I wasn't too enthusiastic about writing this diary. I had second thoughts about revealing my personal and intimate thoughts. A doctor's orders brought about the transcribing of this journal of my life. Out of frustration with me not being able to explain what my symptoms were, the doctor in charge of my initial care told me that I needed to write how I was feeling. So, I began to write down how much pain I was in at any given time or day. I was upset, scared, and hurt. I was seventeen, and confused–I was mad!

All of my notes and my instant reflections were written by hand. This was my way of quickly expressing my thoughts and feelings. I didn't think about it then, but now, I'm glad to see that keeping a journal of as much as I could at the time, had helped me. Whenever I had an inkling to do so, writing gave me a chance to reflect.

To anyone who doesn't know me, this may seem like useless, simple typed scribbles from someone's notepad. Yet now, when a doctor says I need to stop a medication or start a new one, my hands quickly move to my purse. This presents a sort of stop-motion for the doctor as I pull out my journal to show that no disrespect was intended. Now, my physicians smile. And from the pause, my physicians move right back into the recitation of orders as it may be. I still have more of my life's story to tell and this compilation of my first reflections is only the beginning of my journey with lupus.

*"And he said unto her, Daughter, thy faith hath made thee whole; go in peace, and be whole of thy plague."~Mark 5:34 (King James Version)*

## CONTENTS

|   | DEDICATION | iv |
|---|---|---|
|   | ACKNOWLEDGMENTS | v |
|   | PREFACE | vi |
|   | INTRODUCTION | vii |
| 1 | ACCEPTANCE | 1 |
| 2 | DENIAL | 8 |
| 3 | HEADACHES | 16 |
| 4 | MANAGING | 23 |
| 5 | SURVIVAL | 29 |
| 6 | REMISSION | 34 |
| 7 | ADJUST | 40 |
|   | GLOSSARY | 48 |
|   | ABOUT THE AUTHOR | 52 |

# 1

## ACCEPTANCE

During this time, I was in my last year of high school. While all my friends were enjoying fun activities, I was homebound for my entire senior year. And worst of all, my hair was falling out for no reason at all. Scabs formed on the top of my head. I had a high fever that I couldn't explain. I felt weak all the time. At times, I couldn't even pick up a glass of water. My skin was constantly dry. Patches of dry skin could not be remedied with anything I tried. My mother would have to help me bathe and dress myself. The many tests I had to take seemed insurmountable.

The various physicians I went to see did not know what was wrong with me. They diagnosed me with various illnesses. Each doctor's appointment awarded me a new Girl Scout badge. After various different appointments, I was said to have had rheumatoid arthritis, the flu, pneumonia, and mononucleosis. I was frustrated and confused. And all of the medicine I had to take made me feel like a walking guinea pig. A patient physician finally diagnosed me with lupus. At the insistence of this doctor, I started jotting down short notes in a little spiral notebook. No particular format, no structure to sentences were used, because there was no structure to my thoughts. I was attempting to accept my diagnosis.

### Thursday, October 7, 1993
Diagnosed with Systemic Lupus Erythematous- SLE; also known as lupus.

### Tuesday, April 19, 1994
Increase to 60mg Prednisone
1 Plaquenil, 200mg
1 Vasotec, 10mg
3 Zantac, 150mg
Start Carafate, 500mg
Chest pain started 4:30 p.m. along with headaches (constant)

### Wednesday, April 20, 1994
8:00 p.m., headaches. 2:00 p.m., 5:00 p.m., and 1:00 a.m., headaches.
Still severe pain in legs, and feeling of fever in knees and ankles.

### Thursday, April 21, 1994
Took medicine, awoke suddenly with excruciating chest and leg pains; actually feeling pain all over.
Headaches have been coming and going; got stuck in the back of my head.
Took second dose of Prednisone at lunch. Pain still in legs, chest, and head at 8:58 p.m.

### Friday, April 22, 1994
Awoke with chest and leg pains; took medicine in morning
Evening time headache with BP (Blood Pressure) 113/62; pulse 66.

## Saturday, April 23, 1994
7:10 a.m., woke with chest pains and headaches; took Carafate.

## Sunday, April 24, 1994
Chest pains; night chest pains
Legs hurting, light headaches came and went

## Monday, April 25, 1994, Morning
Light headaches in morning
Chest hurts after medicine at 10:45 a.m.

## Monday, April 25, 1994, Evening
I was sitting on my bed, reaching high as I tried to get my sweatpants when West, my boyfriend, saw me about to fall. I had already said that "if I fall, you better catch me," to which he replied, "You know what they say, the best way to fall, is to fall in love…"

My dad spoke at church about love and referenced John 15:15. "The only way you would hurt my feelings is if you tell me you are dead, and I kick you and you move." –Funniest thing I ever heard.

## Tuesday, April 26, 1994
Headaches in the morning time; chest pains

## Wednesday, April 27, 1994
Same old, same old. More headaches and bad pain in legs, swelling in knees and ankles– I JUST FEEL BAD TODAY
Sore throat, chest and leg pains, and a bad headache.
1:00 a.m. – my stomach feels bloated and it hurts. I feel like I'm going to throw up, I'm shaky. 1:30 a.m., I think I'll go to sleep..

Diary of a MAD Lupus Patient         J. H. Johnson

**Thursday, April 28, 1994**
6:40 a.m., took Carafate
Stomach hurts and head feels a little sick, and my chest hurts.

**Friday, April 29, 1994**
Chest pains. Legs hurt. Small headaches

**Saturday, April 30, 1994**
Ate a pinch of salt with my food today. I got sick! My head was hurting so bad and I felt like vomiting.

**Sunday, May 1, 1994**
Headaches, slight stomach pains. Overall sick feeling.

**Monday, May 2, 1994**
Headaches until I don't know when, after I took Carafate, my stomach started hurting and did not stop after eating.
Same pain in legs with fever in knees and ankles.

**Tuesday, May 3, 1994**
Down to 40mg of Prednisone
Headaches remain with continuing stomach pain.

**Wednesday, May 4, 1994**
Headaches, both legs with fever and burning sensations.
Stomach pain, minor chest pains.
I felt nauseous all day and throughout the night.

**Thursday, May 5, 1994**
Horrible pain in legs, knees, and thighs, with burning sensations again.
Felt sick all day, with more headaches.

**Friday, May 6, 1994**
Chest pains again, but my legs are not burning, thankfully.
Headaches, hands shaking; vomiting rest of the day.

**Saturday, May 7, 1994**
Birthday girl headaches, nauseous feeling with stomach pains for the remainder of the day.

**Sunday, May 8, 1994**
Headaches; vomiting at 11:00 a.m.

**Monday, May 9, 1994**
10:30 a.m., pain in my chest hurts; both legs are in pain.
Headache is still here and I feel like I constantly need to vomit.

**Tuesday, May 10, 1994**
Down to 30mg Prednisone
I am figuring out that my stomach hurts when I take Carafate (must remember). Headache, chest hurts little, and fever in legs and ankles.

**Wednesday, May 11, 1994**
Headaches, stomach pains.
No fever.

Diary of a MAD Lupus Patient          J. H. Johnson

**Thursday, May 12, 1994**
Chest hurts (as usual after I take Carafate)
4:00 a.m., chest hurting still; took other medicine.
Headache all day, stomach pains.
10:00 p.m., big headache and fever in hand.
More vomiting, overall feeling sick.

**Friday, May 13, 1994**
Headaches continue, chest pains continue, and
yes, I feel like I need to vomit.

**Saturday, May 14, 1994**
Headaches, legs hurt– extra bad.

**Sunday, May 15, 1994**
Morning headaches, bad pain in legs, and more stomach pains.

**Monday, May 16, 1994**
Headaches, stomach pains, queasy feeling

**Tuesday, May 17, 1994**
Stomach hurts when I take Carafate
Headaches, fever in knees and ankles, and again with the queasy feeling in the late evening.

Diary of a MAD Lupus Patient                    Acceptance

**Wednesday, May 18, 1994**
Stop Carafate.
Down to two Zantacs a day
Take Tylenol for pain.

**Sunday, May 22, 1994, Evening**
What are these pains that come and go? My chest pains come and go. I had chest pains before and after being with West. Was it the night air the day before, or is it just part of the disease? The pains and headaches I'm having now make me paranoid to a high point. The swelling I have is a big curiosity. My wrists show my true figure, and then they swell on outward from the middle to my arm. My hands are spotty red and swollen, along with my face and eyes.

**Friday, May 27, 1994**
Last couple of days had bad headaches and stomach pains. I am still on 30mg of Prednisone and off of the Carafate. I have a pain in my side today, and I am very weak and tired. I went shopping. I walked enough, but I always feel bloated. My legs are always in pain, and they have been hurting worse lately.

**Sunday, May 29, 1994**
Busy day today. I had pains in my side and a "come and go" headache. Other than that, today was a good day with West. We went to Augusta for the whole day, looking and walking and shopping and eating. I experienced a nauseous feeling all day though.

**Monday, May 30, 1994, Memorial Day**
Vomiting, headaches, severe pain in legs; went out with West. I think this pain will never go away– I know it's not all in my mind, and I don't make it out to be worse than it is. But I know it is worse than it should be. I'm trying to be patient.

# 2

## DENIAL

Going from acceptance to denial was probably not a good sign. All of my blood tests proved otherwise. My white blood cell count continued to be low. This was a symptom of lupus, yet the fatigue, ease of bruising, and susceptibility of infection are also symptoms of other diseases. The pain would get so unbearable at times, that I declared to everyone I knew that it couldn't be this thing called lupus.

My joints, my head, my stomach, my muscles, and my everything would hurt! I was constantly nursing my muscle pain. It just had to be something worse, something awful. But what else could it be? I slowly came to accept the reality that lupus, and everything that came with it, was not going away. I began to write a little more and accept a little less.

Diary of a MAD Lupus Patient — Denial

**Tuesday, May 31, 1994**
God bless, I'm still alive! Two days before graduation. My headaches are still constant. The pain in my legs still has not ceased, even with prayer. I'm trying though. Medicine is aggravating, but patience is better, and a must.

**Thursday, June 2, 1994**
I ask myself, why me? The emotions, the pain, why me? Do I deserve this? Is it all in my mind? No, it's just part of life. I've learned today that God sends us through trials and tribulations in order to make us stronger through Christ. He is The Lord.

**Friday, June 3, 1994**
Graduation day– I don't care about pain!

**Sunday, June 5, 1994**
My hands are sore and swollen between my knuckles on the back of my hand. I've had headaches come and go, and pain in my stomach and side. My legs hurt extra bad without use of the walking cane. I'm still trying though.

**Tuesday, June 7, 1994**
The pains never cease, just as I cease to understand them. My stomach hurts when food enters and exits– worse when in, though. My legs refuse to rest; yet the pain does not rest either. I exercised on the skier, yet no sign of relief or relaxation. I know it's not in my mind and my mind knows that the pain is there.

Diary of a MAD Lupus Patient                J. H. Johnson

## Wednesday, June 8, 1994
The family went to Myrtle Beach for the day. We got back at 3:00 a.m.; I walked a lot and rested in between. I think I'm too fat. My head has been hurting all day. Pain in legs as usual— worse after standing for a long time. Fever in very swollen ankles and knees.

## Friday, June 10, 1994
Pain in left side 1:00 a.m. Headache; took Tylenol but not much of a change even though I took a nap. Thankfully, the headache was gone in the afternoon.

## Saturday, June 11, 1994
Went to Myrtle Beach, with friends. I had pain and a headache as usual, but we walked the Boardwalk.

## Sunday, June 12, 1994
Stomach hurts, but after dinner it began to hurt worse. I am swollen all over. Fever in ankles and knees; feel very sick.

## Monday, June 13, 1994
Chest was hurting off and on. Legs hurt. Don't mind much, I am staying out of the sun because my head didn't hurt until I went out outside.

## Friday, June 17, 1994
Chest was hurting Thursday afternoon and night. It came and went. Chest hurting today along with the constant headaches that come and go. I travel and exercise a little and yet, I still feel pain. I have been doing my own therapy on my legs and exercising, yet no change. Just pain. Stomach pain still comes and goes. And maybe it will stop one day. Foot swollen near big toe. Took a bite of my food and stomach started hurting; I think because I took Zantac early. Vomiting and headaches.

Diary of a MAD Lupus Patient	Denial

### Sunday, June 19, 1994
Father's Day – Church
Nightfall – movies – wolf! That's how I feel. I feel like my illness is playing wolf with me. One minute I feel okay, the next I don't. Headaches – cold – legs ache. Side hurt. Bedtime – 12:30 a.m.

### Tuesday, June 21, 1994
Legs hurt considerably. Headaches over the past couple of days. Stomach regular, hands still having problems off and on.

### Wednesday, June 22, 1994
Woke up with chest problems; pains. Headaches off and on, stomach pain as usual. Legs were feverish and hurting in spurts. Side hurts on left.

### Saturday, June 25, 1994
Major headache while I was out with West, I ignored it though. I felt like I needed to vomit because I didn't take my second Zantac in time. My hands started bothering me some. I feel like my memory is making me paranoid– losing it! Stomach pains. Tired because I have been like the energizer bunny; I need to stop and rest.

### Sunday, June 26, 1994
Pain in left side. Headaches while in sun. Swollen, feverish knees. West came over. I noticed when it hurts, I have gas and it makes a pulse in my side.

### Wednesday, June 29, 1994
Now taking 25 mg of prednisone. Dr. Jerry says she refuses to sign disability papers because she feels this would affect me mentally. I have too good of a future. I feel differently. She said I can take her to court! Time and pain will tell. I won't let it stop me. I'll make it. Nothing

more for me to do now, God help me! I will try and see another doctor for a second opinion. I have the right to be upset,; I understand the potential I may have, but what about the money needed to aid me through the college years? I don't plan to sit on a check all my life. It would only be a supplement. I am so worried. I pray and pray that God will help us financially. The answer to this prayer will be "yes," or, "no," but, I think it will be alright.

### Thursday, June 30, 1994

I thought I had problems before, but they could never compare to now. Tears. I thought I was crying tears of pain, but those were not tears of pain. No, no! Pain is now! The tears now are for pain and sorrow, not only for me, but also for the world. When I cry, my heart is bleeding through my eyes, chest pains, probably from burning in legs for some God given reason, I don't know, I just don't know anymore! My side was hurting from gas or something. My mind was moving from curiosity to anything involving emotions to patience…ugh!

### Friday, July 1, 1994

I had two dreams. One composed of large grey stones falling upon me as I ran away. Another was of my cousin. She had a pocket or kitchen knife and I had a long sword. She killed a white dog and me. I don't understand them and I choose not to remember, but everything will be ok.

### Monday, July 4, 1994

Head begins to ache when I walk out in the sun. Severe pain in left side, all day. Legs hurt extremely bad. West and I went out from house to house visiting. I spent the night with him and I enjoyed myself. My legs shook bad. I wonder why the pain insists on coming? Well, let it come. As long as it continues, so will I. And when it stops I'll keep on going even further.

Diary of a MAD Lupus Patient                                    Denial

### Wednesday, July 6, 1994
My knees hurt extra bad today. Stomach pains stretched on until after dinner. I'll take my second Zantac later on tonight. I wonder how long I am going to live. Just how long I will be able to handle this....this pain and curiosity. I hope everything will be okay. Time will tell my story. And pain will become a part of me. Live life as you make it yourself, don't let life make you.

### Saturday, July 9, 1994
2:00 a.m. We had a yard sale today, I am tired, my chest hurts, and here are sharp pains in both legs. I had to push myself to go out with West, I will live though. Ok, God bless Me.

### Sunday, July 10, 1994
Everything persists, even on a Sunday, especially on a Sunday after a busy day like Saturday. I have to keep on going. I'll rest when it's time to rest. Thanks be to the Lord, I'm going.

### Tuesday, July 12, 1994
Lupus is such a curious and aggravating disease. I'll live though. My chest hurts. Took two Good Sense powders for pain at 11:45 p.m.

### Thursday, July 14, 1994
My chest has been hurting lately. But I'll live. I get my allergy shots this month. Headaches too! Took two Good Sense pain relievers. Stomach hurts and vomiting. 2:30 a.m. West came by after work.

### Friday, July 15, 1994
I have never had such a tiresome day. My chest hurts the worst and I almost couldn't breathe as my mouth frothed from lack of water. I felt tired, so tired. At midnight I took two pain relievers and my second Zantac. My left side was also hurting. God bless!

Diary of a MAD Lupus Patient                    J. H. Johnson

### Sunday, July 17, 1994
Headache, vomiting, gas. Took second Zantac late– possible reason, but have had gas lately. It's now close to midnight.; took three Good Sense powders for pain. Goodnight.

### Monday, July 18, 1994
My chest started hurting bad around 8:00 p.m. My legs never let up. Headaches are quickies. Life is short, so I will live it as well as I can. Love ya, God, and thank you.

### Tuesday, July 19, 1994
Sick, very sick. Left side hurts. Up all night– 4:00 a.m., felt like vomiting. Will be okay, I guess. Thank you, Jesus.

### Wednesday, July 20, 1994
Feeling tired. Chest hurting at 11:00 p.m. I went to bed at 9:00 p.m. Guess I'll wait up for West. Did I ever mention that I belch a lot?

### Thursday, July 21, 1994
Went to S.T.E.P. dinner until 10:00 p.m. Charlotte paid– what a nice gesture; I enjoyed myself. Had a headache and severe leg pains. It's ok, I will be all right. Left foot has been hurting, like it's burning inside. Thank you, Jesus.

### Friday, July 22, 1994
My chest was hurting all day. Had a headache and pain in lower left side again. God bless.

## Saturday, July 23, 1994

Chest hurts. Legs hurt extra bad. Went out with West. Forgot second doses of medications for stomach; left side area and head are also in pain. God bless.

## Wednesday, July 27, 1994

I just returned from my first night back from my aunts' place. One of my aunts went to Washington, D.C., for a few days, so I stayed with the other. During my shower, my left leg stung very sharply. West came over for a while. I don't like to tell mama every pain I get. God bless.

## Sunday, July 31, 1994

I haven't been drinking any milk, but I have been taking calcium supplements. I have that pain in my left side and still on both of my hips and kidney area. Headaches.

# 3

## HEADACHES

At first, dealing with pain was not my strong suit. It was a headache to have to accept the fact that the pain may go away in a few minutes or not for a few days. But, I was starting my first year of college and either had to deal with the pain or else. I wasn't interested in the "or else" part of my thoughts. I knew I could do this. I could make it through my first year of college. I had made it this far, why would I give up now. I had read as many books I could get my hands on about pain management and being careful with taking medicine. But who was I kidding. I was my own headache. I was stubborn. I was stubborn enough to fight through the pain and the inconveniences that lupus afforded me.

I felt like I had already spent the beginning of my strength to adjust. Scheduling doctor appointments and numerous medical tests around my homebound school assignments was exhausting. I was adjusting to so many things that it was just a headache to think about more than one thing at a time.

## Wednesday, August 3, 1994
Today I have a headache. My face is awfully swollen. I have no appetite. I took my medicine late. But should that matter? West came over and gave me a kiss. Love him much!

## Saturday, August 6, 1994
Starting 20 mg of Prednisone. I'm at Myrtle Beach, having fun! Thank you, Jesus!

## Thursday, August 18, 1994
Headaches, chest pain. Dr. Jerry said wait a couple of weeks and go down to 15mg of Prednisone. I guess that's why my period came back. God bless.

## Friday, August 19, 1994
The last Friday before school starts. Took Tylenol, voice sounds hoarse. My chest hurts really bad and my fatigue has come sooner than usual. It's been a long summer. When school starts I'll miss West. I hope I'll be blessed some more. Thank you, Jesus.

## Saturday, August 20, 1994
Severe pain on my left side. Nauseous feeling all day and night. Took two Tylenol.

## Wednesday, August 24, 1994
I wonder sometimes about the pain. Is it the pain in my feet? Is it the pain in my legs? Knees? Or the pain in my abdomen and stomach? Is it the pain in my chest? Or is it the pain in my head? In my heart? Yes. Something hurts so badly in my heart and head. Sadness, pain, aggravation and irritation. God will bless me. Thank you, Jesus. I'm already blessed. I will soon be able to rest from this pain.

# Diary of a MAD Lupus Patient    J. H. Johnson

**Friday, August 26, 1994**
I forgot until this evening when I was feeling very sick and painful all over–I started taking 15mg of Prednisone yesterday, Thursday. God, bless me, I'm sick.

**Tuesday, September 6, 1994**
Labor day weekend; I walked a lot without my cane, God bless. But all night my legs pained. I had to force myself to sleep. School was alright today. West started a new job. I didn't get to see him on my break. I miss him and love him. God bless his soul. May one day Jalen, my little brother, speak! Thank you, Jesus!

**Friday, September 9, 1994**
I wonder when I will get better. I wonder if I will ever get better. And I wonder. I guess I'll be okay. I know the Lord is looking down upon me. I know he loves me. I'm tired Lord. I'm selfish now. I'm scared. Please forgive me. Please watch over me. Thank you, Lord, thank you. God bless…success in the future.

**Saturday, September 10, 1994**
I went down to 10 mg of Prednisone. I had a sharp pain by my heart that made me cry while I was with West in Athens today. I swear, I'm still wondering about this disease. God bless.

**Friday, September 23, 1994**
Big step! I went down to 5mg of Prednisone! I only took 5mg this morning and now my legs are hurting bad.

**Saturday, September 24, 1994**
Still on 5mg of Prednisone. Headaches bad all day. Took five Tylenols! Sick as a dog; scared and in pain. May God bless me. West put me to bed. God bless him for understanding. Love is love.

### Sunday, October 2, 1994
I had to go up back to 10 mg of Prednisone. My hands were killing me. God, please take away my pain and illnesses. God bless.

### Thursday, October 20, 1994
Dr. appointment at 9:00 a.m. Start taking 1½ amount of Plaquenil. CT scan is normal, yet pains persist. I do not understand. The higher dosage of Plaquenil is supposed to alleviate some of the pain.

### Thursday, October 27, 1994
Everybody has problems but nobody thinks I do. My friends call me and unload their problems, but I seem to never have a problem to them. Anyway, I would prefer not to bore them with the details. Only God knows my pain and worries. God bless.

### Saturday, November 5, 1994
The bottle of Lecithin says take 4 tablespoons 3 times daily. But I don't want to experience so much at one time. So I only took two with my medicine this morning and my legs went blank! I am limping hard. My bottom lip is swollen –but I think that it was the orange juice I drunk last night because it had swollen up last night. My mouth hurts from the dentist cleaning too.

### Tuesday, November 8, 1994
I'm going to get a treadmill. Non-electric. I'm going to get better. This Christmas will be better than last. Wow! One year with lupus. October 7, 1993- October 7, 1994. I'm blessed to be here. Don't ever forget where you came from.

Diary of a MAD Lupus Patient            J. H. Johnson

### Thursday, November 10, 1994
9:05 a.m., before school, my left knee hurts bad, causing a limp. I've already had taken my medicine. I hope the Lord will take away the pain. Please bless me some more. Forgive all my sins, Lord. And please strike this illness with your might. Amen.

### Friday, November 11, 1994
Although the pain proceeds, I proceed with it. My hands are not a good feeling to awaken to. Even though I have had my flu shot, I still feel achy and a little icky with this lupus. Alli and Dean were in a wreck; the baby is fine but Alli got a small knot on her head. Everybody is fine. My legs have thickened up. My legs hurts bad, like I have a blood clot or something near my ankles and in my knees. They felt like this while I was with my aunts, Eva and Ida. They both smoke heavily. God bless them. I got good exercise today…standing by the sofa.

### Monday, November 14, 1994
Sometimes, I just want to quit. Stop in my tracks and forget it. The pain in the morning is the worst. It makes you wonder if you should be thankful for waking up– I am, but I'm silently suffering. I don't complain too much. Nobody knows but God and me. West, my second heart, doesn't even know. But he soothes me when he says, "I know, I know." Keep exercising, girl! In blessings.

### Tuesday, November 15, 1994
Not a very good day. I missed my Spanish Class. I was feeling bad. I knew it when I couldn't get out of bed this morning. God please give me strength. I practically willed myself to make it to the college to do my part. But someone else wasn't ready. Maybe God didn't want me to push it. Thank you, Jesus. Headaches, bad- very bad. Tiresome-so tiresome.

### Wednesday, November 16, 1994
Coughing and headaches continue. Feel really bad. Will take Tylenol tonight. Goodnight.

### Sunday, November 20, 1994
I awoke with a severe cough and chest cold. While in church my eyes were weeping "yellow cold" as fast as I could get it out. I was in so much pain. I took my medicine and vitamins. I hope I will make it through exams. West and I are supposed to go out, but I am so tired and in so much pain. Wonderful sermon, Daddy, God forgives!

### Saturday, December 3, 1994
I feel like I am going to vomit. I have had migraines since November 24: I feel nauseated, sick, and weak. Chest pain and a little shortness of breath, too. God please watch over me. God bless. Thank you, Lord Jesus.

### Sunday, December 4, 1994
Sometimes, I wonder if I am going to make it. My whole body is stiff and in pain. My ankles are still swollen, my knees are swollen and feel hot to the touch, feverish almost. My hands will not work. My left hand is the stiffest of all. My head is beating like a bass drum. I can hardly walk. I wonder if it is the weather or if it's just me? Finals are next week, so I pray it's just the weather.

### Monday, December 12, 1994
My hands ... the things I have used for so long are suffering so much. They hurt so much. My hands and feet, since December 10, have been hurting. So tender and sore around the ankle and knuckles. The pain doesn't seem to go away. It stays as though to keep me complaining. It lets me know it is there. Can it be the stress from exams or the stress from lupus? West is so patient and loving. This spirit keeps me going.

My family and the things I want for them keep me going too. God bless.

**Saturday, December 17, 1994**
I don't think there is enough paper in the world to write down all the pain I have. May God continue to help me arise in the mornings and may the Good God bless away the pain . . . the pain that hurts so badly.

**Monday, December 19, 1994**
More pain than you can imagine, but what person can imagine pain? The mornings are the worst. When you try to tell someone, they do not understand or they figure it's your problem. Silently suffering or suffering silently, either way it's my life. I smile up towards Jesus and ask him to come bring my medicine to my room. Lord, give me the strength to depend on you and myself. Thank you, Jesus.

# 4

## *MANAGING*

My life has already changed with the onset of a chronic illness. I had to realize that I could not do everything and anything the same. I felt like there were extra steps I had to take to manage my life. Each experience was for the better. Yet, I hadn't realized that all I needed to experience was not complete. Just getting out of bed most mornings required mental strategy. I felt as though life was taking me in circles. I was going back and forth to the doctor and up and down on doses of my medication. And I didn't have a problem with the cliché of pain or no gain. It didn't take a moment for me to gain, while experiencing pain.

Managing a new lifestyle that is forced on you can be quite overwhelming. Lupus was not happy having me as a boss. I did the best I could with what I had. All of my thoughts, purpose, and strength came from my faith.

### Thursday, January 26, 1995
Back pains since yesterday; left hand and foot hurt badly. Pains have been as steady since last reported. God bless, good night.

### Friday, March 3, 1995
Today, I told the doctor about my hell the last couple of days. I wrote the pain down on my pocket calendar; I don't think she understands what I go through. Well, anyway, I am to be off the Zantac within a month– I'm taking the last bit this month. But my pains have been steady.

### Wednesday, March 22, 1995
Yet another one of my hand problems; my left hand hurts so bad tonight.

### Sunday, March 26, 1995
8:25 p.m.,The pain is so bad, help me Jesus.

### Tuesday, March 28, 1995
Did I ever mention that the pain is excruciating in the morning time? It takes so much for me to get out of the bed. It usually eases up later in the evening, but sometimes it doesn't bother. It's lazy pain; pain that sits wherever it wants and only moves to turn the channel– assuming that it has cable. It can switch to any station it pleases. Humph! I'm the houseguest, but does it ask me what I want to watch? No!

### Sunday, April 16, 1995, Easter
This lupus is driving me crazy. I walked the Riverwalk last night with Pookie, and I left the Riverwalk in pain, thinking it would go away. I woke up still in pain. The stiffness in my hands and feet feel like they are getting worse every day. I'm so tired of this thing. I start summer school next month. I figure, why stop school if lupus ain't gonna' stop coming? If only they knew how hard it is to hold a pencil.

### Thursday, May 4, 1995

I went to see Dr. Jerry; my hemoglobin is a little low so she went back up on the Prednisone to 20 mg every other day. I think it's also because of the pain and other stuff I have been having lately. I have had chest pains and my knees and feet hurting more at night. I get so tired and sleepy too quickly. I want to keep doing what I'm doing, but my eyes and body just will not let me. My hand hurts so bad from last night. During this morning's exam, I had to pause and stretch it. I often massage my hands in class anyway. The pain is so bad. I cried myself to sleep last night–all alone with my heating pad.

### Monday, May 15, 1995

I have pain, but no one seems to care. West is being real sweet. I have been able to walk with him without the cane once in a while. I hope this lasts for a while, but lupus is very tricky. I seem to have the pains bad in the morning but worse in the evening. My hands and knees hurt. God, bless me.

### Friday, May 19, 1995

I had to see Dr. Zwerland, my allergy doctor, today. He wants me to come off the Hismanal within three months. First, take one, every other day for a month, then just twice per week. I hate all this medicine and shots. I've never felt comfortable with doctors' attitudes. It seems as though the nurses are the life of the visits. Anyway, I hope I'll be well some day. My hands and fingers are hurting. It is rainy weather; so I guess my lupus will act up a little.

### Saturday, May 20, 1995

I'm having pain in my shoulder like I had when I first started out. My voice is low, and I feel really stressed. I am doing things to keep me busy, like talking and walking, but I still feel terrible. I took some vitamins and two Advil, but they hardly worked. I might go back to Tylenol.

### Wednesday, May 24, 1995
I was taking a shower this morning, because I thought the warm water would help my hands and arms. My left arm was hurting really bad along with my hands. The shower helped a little except I got a sharp pain in my chest under my left breast. I don't know what it was, but it scared me. This whole disease scares me. My chest has been burning, right in the middle, for the last couple of days. Heartburn, maybe?

### Friday, May 26, 1995
My left elbow has begun hurting and has been swollen pretty bad for the last couple of days. Mama put a warm pack on it, but it still hurts bad to move it certain ways. I was sick today. My voice was gone and my body hurt. I hope to ride to Atlanta with West tomorrow. May God watch over me.

### Monday, May 29, 1995, Memorial Day
It's raining. They say the rain affects the bones– arthritis. It's true! I was feeling okay yesterday, but this rain just hit my hands big time. There are so many superstitions with this arthritis and I feel as though I am experiencing them all. Rain or no rain, I still have pain. Yet, when it rains I feel a little tingling with the pain in my joints.

### Tuesday, May 30, 1995
Today, my left foot was hurting bad. When I think I'm okay, I get hit again. My hands bother me too, but I just keep going anyway. I see things happening around the world, and I thank God for how blessed I am. Lord, I know I'm hurting, but I've got to make it. I've got to make it for my family, my father, and myself. I have put up with this pain for so long that now I am accustomed to it. God, watch over me please. Thank you, Amen! I love you, West!

### Sunday, June 4, 1995

West took me out for some frozen yogurt. I decided to watch my weight again. I was doing fine, but I got a headache, so I took some Tylenol and Aleve before it got bad. My throat has been acting up and my voice has been coming and going. No pain while swallowing though. A little pain in the sides. I can't wait until this lupus goes away. I pray I'll be able to wake one morning without pain. God bless.

### Wednesday, June 14, 1995

My hands hurt a little. I taught Vacation Bible School this week. It's hard to do the crafts and such while your hand hurts. My throat is a little better, but I still get confused with the pain. God bless. Success.

### Friday, June 16, 1995

I haven't been feeling well today. I don't know what it is or, maybe I do. I hope to feel better soon. My hands have been acting up this morning. I have a headache and pain in my feet; I ate only a plum for breakfast with 20mg of Prednisone, maybe that's the problem. I have been taking my vitamins and Tylenol, too.

### Sunday, July 2, 1995

My whole body hurts really bad. I soaked in Epsom Salt in the tub, but my body still hurts. (West wrote this in my diary for me, I love him!)

### Saturday, July 3, 1995

The past week has been very bad. Pain everywhere, even in my throat and head. I have been limping and my hands couldn't even roll up West's car window and I wonder if it is because it has been raining all week. May God take this pain away.

Diary of a MAD Lupus Patient    J. H. Johnson

**Friday, July 14, 1995**
A day before the big beach trip with West, and I have so much pain that I'm scared! My hands and shoulder have been hurting all week– I'm so scared. I have been taking everything I'm supposed to but still, I have pain. God, please watch over me.


**Monday, July 24, 1995**
I'm back…and so is my lupus. It left with me, and it returned with me. Oh well. My hands and knees hurt the worst on the trip. I had a good time though. I took Naproxen (Aleve) with me, but hardly anything works for me. I get so aggravated sometimes. My mood changes every time pain strikes. I keep thinking, if my hands hurt like this during school, I'll have to go through my second year of college with this pain. God, help me.

# 5

## SURVIVAL

"Either live with it, or let it live with you," had become my rule to live by. I told myself I had too much to do and too much to live for. I had to survive lupus. I had to show this wild beast of a disease that it had no control on the path I decided to take, so I worked hard at trying to control my symptoms. Yet the blood work proved that I still had to submit to some of its need to cause chaos in my life. I hated walking through this jungle that lupus created. I wanted to feel a clear path. I wanted to take the path without pain. I wanted out.

At this point, my survival instincts had settled in. If I wanted to survive, I needed a plan of action. I knew it wouldn't be easy, but I had to try. I had to learn how to tame the wild beast. Intertwining lupus and its chores into my schedule required a survival technique.

Diary of a MAD Lupus Patient                    J. H. Johnson

**Tuesday, August 1, 1995**
Lately, my hands have been hurting so bad, I can't even squeeze my hand towel or brush my teeth without straining in the morning and afternoon. I don't understand. It hurts so much. Sometimes, I feel like I'm the only one suffering with all this pain. I know God will bless me. I'm already blessed, but this pain hurts so much. I'll keep going though and tell myself it's all in my mind. I can't even comb my hair! God, forgive.

**Friday, August 4, 1995**
Today, my face has been swollen and I felt like I was going to vomit. I think I'm just tired, so very tired.

**Sunday, August 27, 1995**
The first week of school was rough. My legs and hands never failed to ignore me. I was in a lot of pain. Sometimes, I wonder why I put myself through it. The whole right side of my body ailed me from my head to my foot. I limped from the movies with West at about 6:30 p.m.; I cried. I can't understand how West puts up with me. And I never will understand lupus. Love makes the pain tolerable; love, always.

**Saturday, September 9, 1995**
My chest has been hurting since yesterday. I hope I'm not getting sick again. I'll take something for it right now. Maybe that Naproxen? Other than that, things have been kind of steady. May God continue to bless me, as he has. Thank you, Jesus!

**Monday, September 18, 1995**
This lupus hurts! It started gradually this morning. Then by 10:00 p.m., my feet were hurting and I was limping on my right foot. Oh! I'm so tired of lupus. My hands and back hurt extraordinarily bad. I'm going to go to sleep early.

### Tuesday, September 19, 1995

I have an accounting test today. I am still waking up with pain, in fact, more pain. My lower left side of my back hurts and my feet and hands still bother me. I took two Tylenol and 250 mg of Naproxen last night before bedtime. I guess lupus is winning this game. Yet, I think not.

### Wednesday, October 4, 1995

I'm starting to feel uncomfortable during my doctor appointments. I am now to take 80 mg of aspirin or less, continue taking 400 mg of Plaquenil and keep alternating 20 mg/10 mg of Prednisone. I feel as though the pains are not in my mind, even though I am doing well with my disease. I am not crazy. I am proud of my achievements despite this disease, but I don't need an anti-depressant drug or psychiatrist to tell me. I got my throat test. I go to the ENT (ear, nose, and throat) doctor on October 16. Oh, I got my flu shot too!

### Thursday, October 5, 1995

The doctor says she has done what she can do for now. I know my swelling, fever, and inflammation don't show signs around her, but I'd like for her to jump in my shoes for one night into the morning. Yes, I know I'm an extraordinary patient. When pain hits, I refuse to stay still. I have a life to live, and I'm going to live it. The Lord is bringing me closer to him with everyday of my suffering. What Tylenol and Aleve can't do (which isn't much) the Good Lord will do. I don't see or understand how psychological medicine is going to manage my pains. One, I don't need an anti-depressive drug; because I sleep well and am not depressed. And two, I don't need a psychiatrist or psychologist; because I have too many kinds of mind bogglers in my family. They just don't understand and love me. God bless.

### Tuesday, October 10, 1995
I'm so tired of pain. Just when I think I'm doing fine I get hit in the hand, knee, leg, foot, or head, etc... I don't need a psychiatrist for pain management. I need one to handle my pain for me. Anyway, my left hand is killing me. I am taking a Naproxen before I sleep tonight. Hopefully, I'll wake up feeling a little better.

### Monday, October 16, 1995
I went to the Ear, Nose and Throat doctor today. I left crying and frustrated. I was put back on Zantac in order to control the reflux of acid that they claim is causing the puffiness in my throat. Also, I am to go to a speech therapist to learn vocal hygiene. Huh? I'm so tired of all this crap. I am going to continue to pray and have faith in the Lord. Thank you, Lord.

### Wednesday, October 25, 1995
Today, I saw the vocal hygienist. She gave me a worksheet to go by and study. I am to learn vocal techniques to try to get rid of the puffiness and swelling on my vocal cords. I'm a little frightened that I may have to have them removed surgically. I am to see her for six weeks. I'm going to pray and hope that I don't have to go through any more of this. I'm tired!

### Saturday, October 28, 1995
I can hold a pencil. I had a lot of studying to do. But I felt bad and my right shoulder, was hurting real bad. I took a long nap and overslept into my study time. Anyway, I felt bad the whole morning. Later on I took two Aleve. I felt better around five o'clock. West took me out, and I enjoyed myself. God bless me.

### Thursday, November 2, 1995
I am so tired of this pain, but I pray that it will cease. Tonight I continue my vocal hygiene therapy and the exercises with that. My left foot, stomach, and head are hurting real bad. With lupus, and voice therapy, I have had it. I hope to handle this pain as best as I can. May God watch over me and bless me.

### Friday, November 3, 1995
My ears have been ringing for two days now, off and on. I have not been feeling too well lately. It's probably the weather. My stiffness is bad and my concentration is off. Headaches have been hovering over me lately, also. I'll try not to concentrate too hard. God knows.

### Saturday, November 4, 1995
My throat is getting worse! It hurts, bad!

### Sunday, November 5, 1995
I don't know what it is about my throat, and my left side, the one I have been complaining about for the longest– the pain is off and on. But when it hurts, it hurts. Anyway, I hope I don't have a bad case of the sore throat—any hurting throat is a bad throat to use for swallowing. Lupus is hurting me all over my body. I am taking strong medicines hoping they'll kill it by tomorrow. I have got to go to class tomorrow. Lord knows I do!

### Tuesday, November 7, 1995
I have been so sore lately. My entire body hurts like one whole pain. I plan to get seen about this side; in the meantime I'm drinking more water and taking too many pain pills. I can't help it, I have to go to these last few weeks of class. I hope I am not too sick. May God watch over me. I feel so terrible–from my throat, to my head, to my feet, I hurt.

# 6

## *REMISSION*

By the time I acknowledged lupus and the fact that it was not going away, I thought I had it under control. Although I did not know it at the time, the previous months proved to be only a settling phase. The highpoint of my illness was not as apparent as it was when my illness was in remission. My doctor told me that my C-Reactive Protein (CRP) levels were low. This meant, by the test standards, that my lupus wasn't as active as it had been before. It was odd, I thought. Why was I experiencing so much physical turmoil if my lupus was supposed to be in this shell called remission?

This time in my life was the re-admittance of a lupus flare. I had had enough of the back and forth and ups and downs; I needed to re-trace my steps and review my needs. I had learned that symptoms from a chronic illness are in remission when they are not active. Yet, I knew my body was experiencing inflammation. I felt it all over. I was still confused. I needed to learn exactly what my symptoms were doing. The CRP test had to be wrong.

### Wednesday, June 19, 1996
Notes from doctor's appointment: 30 mg of Prednisone a day until Sunday. Then, take 30 mg Monday, Wednesday, Friday, and Sunday. Take 15mg on Tuesday, Thursday, and Saturday. Stop Disalcid. Take Naproxen only if you have pain. Take Carafate. Build hemoglobin up. Call next Wednesday to tell how you are doing. Check blood pressure.

### Wednesday, July 17, 1996
Notes from doctor's appointment: Take 10 mg Prednisone on Tuesday, Thursday, and Saturday. Take 30 mg on Monday, Wednesday, Friday, and Sunday. In three weeks, if I feel good, take 10 mg Tuesday, Thursday, and Saturday. Take 25 mg Monday, Wednesday, Friday, and Sunday. Start Carafate, once a day in the evening. If she does not call, do the changes. Watch throat. Continue Plaquenil as I have been.

### Thursday, August 29, 1996
In one month, take 25 mg of Prednisone on Monday, Wednesday, Friday, and Sunday. Take 5 mg on Tuesday, Thursday, and Saturday. Diet: Tuna for calcium; less salt; get some supportive shoes; drink fluids, see eye doctor two times a year for eye exam; get my flu shot next month. If I decide on birth control, use low estrogen only.

### Thursday, October 17, 1996
Weight…watch weight. Birth control. In two weeks, start taking Plaquenil- one in the morning and one-half in the evening. Weaning off of Prednisone. Start 1 and one eighth of Prednisone? I don't know what that means! By the mid–November I am to alternate by taking 20 mg and 5 mg of Prednisone.

Makde eight-week appointment; checked my blood pressure at Wal-Mart because I was having dizziness symptoms and headaches. BP reading on 10/09/96 reads 121/72, pulse 102. On 10/16/96 blood pressure reading is 118/64, pulse 107; second take 111/62, pulse 105.

Diary of a MAD Lupus Patient                    J. H. Johnson

### Tuesday, October 29, 1996
On Thursday, Oct. 30, started taking Plaquenil as directed and today I was laid up with a bad left arm. I have taken so many pain relievers that I believe that I have developed a resistance to them. I go to the Gynecologist on Thursday afternoon.

### Wednesday, November 20, 1996
Office visit with Dr. Jerry, 11:12 a.m,. Notes: Take 5 mg of Prednisone this evening, and then increase to 25 mg/5 mg every other day. If in two days not feeling much better, go up to 25 mg/7.5 mg. Take one Tums every other day. Doc also said that because infections are hidden by steroids, if not feeling any better, go to emergency room.

### Saturday, November 23, 1996
Head still hurting and my body hurts too, especially my hands and arms. After reporting symptoms to my doctor, I will now take a half a tablet of the 5mg Prednisone.

### Monday, November 25, 1996
On 25 mg of Prednisone, my head started hurting, and it has gotten bad now. I'm in bed; it feels like a big migraine. My chest doesn't hurt too badly with it, I just wish it would go away. I took a 325 mg of aspirin. I will take an Excedrin for the first time in a couple of minutes. I hope it works. God bless.

### Thursday, December 19, 1996
Dr. Jerry says 22.5 mg/7.5 mg of Prednisone for now, then in January reduce to 20 mg/7.5 mg. Watch diet, get exercise; watch weight.

### Friday, January 3, 1997
Started taking 20 mg/7.5 mg today. Still with one and a half Plaquenil a day, one Aspirin, and one Tums. Sometimes, I feel like I am going crazy. I see things and feel paranoid– I hope I'm not going crazy...

### Wednesday, January 15, 1997
Chest pains started the same weekend I started Prednisone. Today is the 15th, and they are getting worse, as well as my breathing.

### Wednesday, February 12, 1997
Stay with current dosage of medicine. Start taking Calcium and vitamin D. Start getting more rest and add exercise into your schedule. I saw a dietitian today, again. She stated to stay consistent and watch my diet– the goal is to lose 5 pounds. Make sure to get 400 IU's of vitamin D. Drink plenty of water and don't skip meals. Try to take Centrum Silver.

### Tuesday, February 18, 1997
Today, I experienced weakness and my hands were hurting bad. I could hardly hold onto the steering wheel.

### Friday, February 21, 1997
Today, I felt a little weak. Pain in my chest area, upper left. I took some store brand cold medicine for my slightly stuffy nose and sneezing.

### Friday, February 28, 1997
I have flu-like symptoms. My left knee is hurting, swollen, and feverish. My chest hurts slightly, and I have had to take Tylenol for headaches. I took some store brand Tussin for my cough.

### Tuesday, March 11, 1997
My left foot is swollen and hurts badly; my right hand, also. I feel very tired and weak. I have been standing off and on all day. Trying to fight this pain since it is my spring break, but it hurts so much. Will ask for a chest x-ray as I have had little pains in chest.

### Thursday, March 20, 1997
Today, my chest pains are still here. They were bad yesterday. I had pain in both my chest and head. It's early morning, so I don't know what the rest of the day will bring yet.

Diary of a MAD Lupus Patient          J. H. Johnson

**Friday, March 21, 1997**
Chest pain, dizziness, and fever. I have been taking Tylenol all day long.

**Sunday, March 23, 1997**
Call Friday and let the doctor know how I am doing. Hospital-admitted in. Find out results concerning chickenpox. Had an IV run through me Sunday and Monday with steroids and antibiotics. Next time I feel bad, slow down, rest, and call to avoid this. I took 60 mg of Prednisone Monday 3/24; EKG for heart, and wait for chickenpox results. Change prescription dosage- 40 mg tomorrow for three days, and 30 mg from then on. The doctor will see how I am doing before dropping it lower.

**Saturday, March 29, 1997**
Had a high fever and sweated it out with rest and Tylenol. By the end of the day, I was feeling better and walking around; slight chest pain though.

**Sunday, March 30, 1997, Easter**
Slight chest pain. Took 30 mg of Prednisone starting today. I feel alright, just a little chilled and tired. Tightness in the chest area– Dr. Jerry said to take 10 mg more. Going to hospital.

**Monday, March 31, 1997**
I went to a scheduled emergency room appointment, Dr. Jerry told me to come in. Today I am to take 60 mg of Prednisone. Had an EKG and chest x-rays done because of pain and fever. Tomorrow, take 40 mg Prednisone–20 mg in morning and 20mg in the evenings.

**Wednesday, April 9, 1997**
Dr. Jerry said no travel this weekend because there is fluid around my heart. Take 60 mg of Prednisone all in the morning on the 16th of April. Take 50 mg the following Sunday. Forgot and took 50 mg on following Tuesday morning, April 22. Made an appointment for April 23.

## Wednesday, April 16, 1997
Start 60 mg of Prednisone in morning. Chest pain (4:00 p.m., hard) all day. Feel a little weak and tired, but continued regular activity.

## Friday, April 18, 1997
I took 60 mg of Prednisone in the morning. The acid reflux has been an aggravation. It disturbs my sleep. My burps cause my chest to hurt badly. My legs started hurting today, also. I have chest pains and my head is aching, too. The deeper pain comes and goes. The rest of the time, it just sits there.

## Wednesday, April 23, 1997
One week more on 50 mg, then switch down to 40 mg. Don't wait 'til appointment time if feeling bad. Appointment will be scheduled with cardiologist same day. Slow down; get more rest until fluid calms down. Watch activities and eyes.

# 7

## ADJUST

With a shortness of breath, bag full of medicine, and chest full of pain, I slowed down, a little. I know that my stubbornness and not slowing down earlier in the stages of my diagnosis, may have contributed to the many flares I combated. It was back to short notes and quick reminders for me to keep on the course towards survival. The rainbow of medicines didn't have a pot of golden health at the end. The pot was becoming filled with notes of pain and hopes of change. At this point I didn't care. I could draw my gun as quick as lupus could. I was ready for what lupus wanted to dish out. I was beginning to be less shy about calling the doctor and leaving messages. I didn't mind if I was in pain, I was going to that game. I was going to go that party. I was going to ride to the beach, even if I had to drive myself.

It was becoming apparent that I had to do more than adjust. I had to make sure I wasn't spinning from acceptance and back to denying that I had lupus. I had to accept the fact that lupus is my headache. And in order to survive, I had to be ready for remission, re-admission, and sometimes submission, to the pain. I knew that my lupus symptoms would come and go as they pleased. I was ready to manage that element of lupus. I just had to hang on and adjust to my situation.

## Thursday, May 1, 1997
Started taking 40 mg of Prednisone, all in the morning. Busy day—came home at 2:00 p.m., took two extra strength Tylenol for slight chest pain that has been here all day..

## Friday, May 9, 1997
Headaches, chest hurting again; I have been taking Tylenol and Aspirin. Took an Excedrin at 7:00 p.m.

## Monday, May 12, 1997
Chest still continually hurting.

## Wednesday, May 14, 1997
Went to see Dr. Jerry; instructed me to go up to 60 mg of Prednisone, until further notice. Call on Friday morning.

## Sunday, May 25, 1997
Just came back from Six Flags, had chest pains. I took Tylenol for fever and pains. Got some sleep. Still a little chest pain. I have been taking aspirin for the pains during the school week. I will rest after my test on Tuesday.

## Wednesday, May 28, 1997
Prednisone down to 50 mg (blood work was low). Plaquenil: take one in the morning and one in the evening. Baby aspirin, Tums, and vitamins. Possibly pulmonary testing and chest scan on the day of the cardiologist visit. Bear with the pain, get more rest this summer, and don't push myself. In one year will transfer to University Hospital for care. Carafate in the evening at bedtime. Pulmonary test is done because of concern with pneumonia. Spirometry study required.

Diary of a MAD Lupus Patient    J. H. Johnson

### Wednesday, June 4, 1997
Chest pains in the last two days, maybe because I have been busy. Took two Tylenol and got an extra nap. I feel a little better today.

### Monday, June 9, 1997
Some chest pain before and after walking around the block with my dog, Trey; but worse after. I had ignored my pain Sunday, I was real busy. I probably did too much.

### Sunday, June 15, 1997
I had chest pains off and on all week– it gets harder at the end of the day and not too bad in the morning time, mostly after activity.

### Tuesday, June 24, 1997
Oral thrush started Saturday. I went to med center for Diflucan today– must take for 2 weeks. The chest pain was bad today and but only a little yesterday.

### Saturday, July 5, 1997
Slight chest pain. Took a nap at 7:00 p.m., awoke with pain. Took a regular strength aspirin, going to sleep. The other day had pain, took two Tylenols and pain got milder, but didn't go away completely. Today it was off and on because I went shopping with Mama.

### Monday, July 7, 1997
My chest started hurting around 8:00 p.m. I'm going to take two Tylenol and go to sleep.

### Thursday, July 10, 1997
Chest hurting all day. Got worse around 8:30 p.m. I have been running around, not sure if that's why.

### Wednesday, July 16, 1997
Doctor's appointment. Try heating pad with moist cloth against chest. Try Advil. Might consider coming down on Prednisone after blood work. If not then, will start instructions on a new medication. Bring calcium supplements (vitamins) on next visit. New doctor referral? Dr. Penny Williams will call to schedule.

### Sunday, August 24, 1997
The past couple of days I have had pain in my hips. I can't stand or walk much for any length of time. My chest put me out of commission Saturday. Chest pain and acid reflux is just killing me. I could hardly eat.

### Thursday, August 28, 1997
Dr. Jerry recommends cutting the Prednisone down to 40 mg a day, increase Pepcid, and work on my weight. After visit with Dr. Williams, she says if I'm not sure, to call her for second opinion if I choose to do so. I will be signing a release of information form to her (October 7, 1993,-May 28, 1997).

### Thursday, October 23, 1997
I have had and have been fighting this ingrown toenail for two weeks. Dr. Williams went down on my Prednisone. Dr. Fitte cut my toenail out. I have 10 more days of antibiotics and cutting Prednisone to 2.5 mg a week until my next appointment. All I can say is gee-whiz. Not to mention the problem with money and medicine. I'm over my Medicaid medical limit.

### Thursday, November 20, 1997
Today, the doctor said to go down to 25 mg Prednisone a day. I told her my chest wasn't hurting, but it was. Only last night and today. I figured I'll get over it. I'll start down to 27.5 mg tomorrow. Then, work my way down. I'll keep myself warm too. God bless!

### Friday, November 28, 1997
I threw up just now. It's 1:00 in the morning. I am currently taking 25 mg a day of Prednisone. I hope it's alright. I have not been feeling well lately, but I pray it will pass. I have the heating pad on my chest for the evening. God bless.

### Wednesday, December 3, 1997
My chest is still hurting. I am using the heating pad. I hope it stops soon. Called Dr. Williams, and she said take 25 mg of Prednisone tonight. I'm mad!

### Thursday, December 4, 1997
Due to pain, I am to start taking 40 mg of Prednisone. Take 25 mg of Prednisone in the morning. Take 15 mg of Prednisone in the evening. Take three Plaquenil per day. Alternate nostrils on sinus spray. One nostril per day. Start Caltrate; take twice daily. Get eyes checked soon.

### Tuesday, December 9, 1997
My chest pains woke me up twice last night. I still have some pain just sitting there and a dull headache too.

### Wednesday, December 10, 1997
My chest is still hurting. It woke me up twice last night.

### Friday, December 12, 1997 to Saturday, December 13, 1997
Hospital stay at University Hospital in Georgia. They ran tests on my heart. The doctor let me go home Saturday evening. I was placed back on 50 mg of Prednisone and given some pain medication called Darvocet, or something like that.

### Thursday, December 18, 1997
In one week come down 5 mg to 45 mg of Prednisone. Continue pain medication. Get 48 hours of bed rest. Chest pain is due to Pleurisy caused by the lupus

### Thursday, January 15, 1998
Start 40 mg Prednisone daily and a new stomach medication. I haven't been up to par lately. Real fatigued and achy.

### Wednesday, January 21, 1998
Very sleepy all the time and my hands are real shaky. Goodness knows.

### Thursday, January 22, 1998
My hands have been so shaky lately since I have been taking this extra medication. My nerves are bad. I get dizzy and really sleepy in class. I almost fell asleep driving to school. I feel sick and slightly nauseated.

### Monday, January 26, 1998
I called Dr. Williams and was told to stop taking the Prilosec and Flexeril and start back on the Pepcid, 40 mg, until my next appointment. I still have a little bit of the shakes and pain all over. I guess it's the weather.

### Monday, February 9, 1998
I was out of school last week. I have my doctor's excuse. I still do not feel very well. I'm back on the Flexeril for muscle spasms. Yet, I feel pain all over; my legs feel heavy and my hands are shaky. They aren't steady at all. I get weak and can't stay asleep at night. I took some Pepcid and 40 mg of Mylanta, but they aren't working at all to keep that reflux down. I'll pray that I can sleep tonight. Avascular Necrosis (hips)? Possibility?

Diary of a MAD Lupus Patient                    J. H. Johnson

### Monday, February 9, 1998, Evening
I took a nap at 10:00 p.m. and intended to wake up at 11p.m. to study. I wound up waking up at 11:20 p.m., throwing up again. This one hurt and wouldn't stop. I don't know what doesn't agree with me and my stomach. I pray this lupus away. I'm coughing and sniffing, also.

### Tuesday, February 10, 1998
6:00 a.m., I woke up with my legs hurting real bad. Hope I can go to school.

### Tuesday, March 3, 1998
I woke up about 12:35 a.m. last night, rushing to take the heating pad off my chest. I ran over to the bathroom, and began vomiting again. My stomach is still a little upset this morning. I hope I am not getting too sick again. I hate this feeling! My legs and head have been hurting for the last two weeks. I have been fighting it to the best of my ability.

### Friday, April 4, 1998
Nauseated all day. My legs and hips are still hurting. Dizzy and tired. Awoke at 12:30 a.m. and vomited up my dinner.

### Sunday, April 5, 1998
Nauseated. Acid reflux in the middle of the night. Hips and legs hurt. Stomach aches all day. Headache this evening.

### Monday, April 6, 1998
Dazed all day. Felt bad. Nauseated this evening, more acid reflux. Pain still bad in hip and left knee.

### Tuesday, April 7, 1998

Pain in my hip. Reflux. In the evening, I didn't take all my medicine when I ate. I felt like I was going to throw up. Dizzy and dazed, and can't drive at night. Eyes fuzzy.

### Wednesday, April 8, 1998

I had a bad feeling all day; terribly nauseated, dizzy, and hands were shaking at school. Took nap at home and awoke with nausea and pain. Head feels tight, my stomach hurts. I have a few questions to ask during my next doctor's visit:

Does the nausea have to do with my hip? Am I really borderline diabetic? Why can't I lose this weight? Can I start applying for jobs?

## *GLOSSARY*

**Acetaminophen** - is a pain reliever and a fever reducer used for various purposes and to treat many conditions such as headache, muscle aches, arthritis, backache, toothaches, colds, and fevers.

**Antibodies** - a protein produced by the body's immune system when it detects harmful substances, called antigens (microorganisms such as bacteria, fungi, parasites, and viruses) and chemicals.

**Anti-depressants** – medication prescribed for depression to work to balance some of the natural chemicals in our brains.

**Aspirin** – is used to reduce pain, fever, and inflammation and is sometimes used to treat or prevent heart attacks, strokes, and chest pain.

**Autoimmune Disease** - any disorder in which loss of function or destruction of normal tissue arises from humoral or cellular immune responses to the body's own tissue constituents; may be systemic, as Systemic Lupus Erythematosus, or organ specific, as Thyroiditis.

**Autoimmune Disorder** – a condition produced when antibodies may be produced when the immune system mistakenly considers healthy tissue a harmful substance.

**Avascular Necrosis** - the death of bone tissue due to a lack of blood supply and can lead to tiny breaks in the bone and the bone's eventual collapse.

**Blood Pressure (BP)** - the pressure or tension of the blood within the systemic arteries, maintained by the contraction of the left ventricle, the resistance of the arterioles and capillaries, the elasticity of the arterial walls, as well as the viscosity and volume of the blood; expressed as relative to the ambient atmospheric pressure.

**Calcium** - is necessary for many normal functions of the body, especially bone formation and maintenance and can also bind to other minerals (such as phosphate) to aid in their removal from the body.

**Carafate** - an anti-ulcer medication that works mainly in the lining of the stomach by adhering to ulcer sites and protecting them from acids, enzymes, and bile salts.

**Chronic Fatigue** - a syndrome of persistent, incapacitating weakness or fatigue, accompanied by nonspecific somatic symptoms, lasting at least 6 months, and not attributable to any known cause.

**C-Reactive Protein (CRP)** - a protein in the body that can act as a marker for inflammation.

**CT Scan** - a computed tomography (CT) scan is an imaging method that uses x-rays to create pictures of cross-sections of the body.

**Darvocet** - contains a combination of propoxyphene and acetaminophen; is used to relieve mild to moderate pain with or without fever. Withdrawn from U.S. market in 2010.

**Diflucan** - is an antifungal antibiotic used to prevent fungal infection in people with weak immune systems.

**Disability** – an impairment present from birth, or occurring during a lifetime that may be physical, cognitive, mental, sensory, emotional, developmental, or some combination of these.

**Disalcid** – a drug that works by reducing substances in the body that causes pain, fever, stiffness, and inflammation.

**EKG** – an electrocardiogram (EKG or ECG) is a test that checks for problems with the electrical activity of the heart.

**Epsom salt** – regarded as a natural remedy that has health benefits to include relaxing the nervous system, helping skin problems, soothing back pain, aching limbs, muscle strain, and healing cuts, cold and congestion, and drawing toxins from the body.

**Flexeril** - a muscle relaxant that works by blocking nerve impulses (or pain sensations) that are sent to the brain.

**Hemoglobin** - a protein in red blood cells that carries oxygen.

**Hismanal** – a long-acting and selective oral histamine. Withdrawn from U.S. market in 1999.

**Immune system** - an intricate complex of interrelated cellular, molecular, and genetic components that provides a defense, the immune response, against foreign organisms or substances and aberrant native cells.

**Inflammation** - the body's attempt at self-protection; the aim being to remove harmful stimuli, including damaged cells, irritants, or pathogens and begin the healing process.

**Lecithin** - used to modify the immune system by activating specific and nonspecific defense systems, treating memory disorders such as dementia and Alzheimer's disease, treating gallbladder disease, liver disease, certain types of depression, high cholesterol, anxiety, and certain types of skin disease.

### Diary of a MAD Lupus Patient          J. H. Johnson

**Lupus** - a chronic inflammatory disease that occurs when your body's immune system attacks your own tissues and organs.

**Lupus Foundation of America** - (LFA) is the largest national non-profit voluntary health organization dedicated to finding the causes of and cure for lupus and providing support, services and hope to all people affected by lupus.

**Mononucleosis** (mono) - is a viral infection in which there is an increase of white blood cells that are mononuclear (with a single nucleus).

**Mylanta** - is an over the counter medication used for the treatment of acid reflux, heartburn, and gastro esophageal reflux disease (also known as GERD).

**Naproxen** – a drug that works by reducing hormones that causes inflammation and pain in the body.

**Pepcid** - a histamine-2 blocker that works by decreasing the amount of acid the stomach produces and is used to treat and prevent ulcers in the stomach and intestines.

**Pleurisy** - inflammation of the lining of the lungs and chest (the pleura) that leads to chest pain.

**Pneumonia** - an infection in one or both of the lungs.

**Prednisone** - a dehydrogenated analogue of cortisone with the same actions and uses; must be converted to prednisolone before active; inhibits proliferation of lymphocytes.

**Prilosec** - is used alone or with other medications to treat the backward flow of acid from the stomach causes heartburn.

**Pulmonary test** - tests that measure how well the lungs take in and release air for the body's circulation.

**Rheumatoid Arthritis** - is a chronic inflammatory disorder that typically affects the small joints in your hands and feet.

**Spirometry** - is a test used to diagnose conditions that affect breathing such as how much air is inhaled and exhaled.

**Steroids** - are similar to hormones that adrenal glands produce to fight stress associated with illnesses and injuries and is used reduce inflammation and affect the immune system.

**Stress** - the body's reaction to a change that requires a physical, mental or emotional adjustment or response which can come from any situation, thought, or continuous use of medications.

**Systemic Lupus Erythematosus -** is an autoimmune, inflammatory disease of the connective tissues, chiefly characterized by skin eruptions, joint pain, recurrent pleurisy, and kidney disease; also called lupus.

**Vasotec** - used to treat high blood pressure, congestive heart failure, and a disorder of the ventricles.

**Vitamin D** – is a vitamin used for, but not limited to, treating weak bones, bone pain, bone loss, and preventing low calcium and bone loss in people with kidney failure.

**Vocal Hygienist** – provides guidance on maintaining proper vocal fitness for the vocal chords muscles.

**Zantac** - used to treat and prevent ulcers in the stomach and intestines. It also treats conditions in which the stomach produces too much acid.

## ABOUT THE AUTHOR

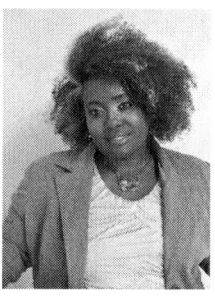

J. H. was diagnosed with Systemic Lupus Erythematosus, known unassumingly as lupus, in early 1993. The beginning of her walk with lupus was painful and confusing. During her senior year in high school, she was placed as a homebound student. This required her to finish her last year of high school education from the confinements of her bedroom. Not discouraged, she completed her senior year of high school with honors. She graduated from the University of South Carolina-Aiken with a bachelor in Business Education, with minors in Marketing and Accounting. J. H. moved on to complete her graduate studies with an Educational Specialist degree from Nova Southeastern University in Computing Technology in Education.

She taught in the K12 public educational system for 7 years. Later in her career, she realized that her true calling was professionally training teachers and administrators. As a professional development facilitator, she travels nationwide to deliver instructional technology based training services. J. H. enjoys her full-time job and treasures the opportunity to meet interesting people every day. As far as she is concerned, there are no dull moments from traveling and training. J. H. is known for her energetic, pom-pom spirit phrases and continues to surprise many when it is discovered that she has been suffering with lupus for almost 20 years.

J. H. continues to share her tidbits of her remarkable journey with lupus on her blog at www.thelupusliar.com. She is the author of several books to include her soon to be released book entitled "Keep Up With Lupus: A Digital Guide." Her continued journey inspires those who know her to keep close to heart, life's ups and downs, happiness and trials. She continues to see a physician regularly. The gift of a healthy life is not often received, yet, the art of loving the life that you have and the health that you can achieve, makes life all the more special. J. H. is indeed, a genuine example of a Lupus Warrior.

Diary of a Mad Lupus Patient
Shortness of Breath
Copyright © 2012 J. H. Johnson
All rights reserved.
ISBN: 0988881055
ISBN-13: 978-0-9888810-5

## Discussion Questions

What possible symptoms supported the diagnosis of lupus?

How is lupus diagnosed?

What other complications were experienced due to the onset of lupus?

Does lupus really cause so much pain on a daily basis?

What are other treatments that could have been prescribed to help with the symptoms?

How is the author doing today?

*Got more questions? Want to find out how J. H. Johnson is doing today? Feel free to email your questions to jhjohnsonbooks@gmail.com.*

*Join the mailing list for Diary of a Mad Lupus Patient 2: Moving Forward with Faith.*